A DAILY
DOSE OF
WOMEN'S
WISDOM

ALSO BY DR CHRISTIANE NORTHRUP

Books

Making Life Easy

Goddesses Never Age

Mother-Daughter Wisdom

The Secret Pleasures of Menopause

The Secret Pleasures of Menopause Playbook

The Wisdom of Menopause

The Wisdom of Menopause Journal

Women's Bodies, Women's Wisdom

Beautiful Girl

Miscellaneous

Women's Bodies, Women's Wisdom Oracle Cards

Audio Programs

Goddesses Never Age

Creating Health

The Empowering Women Gift Collection (with Louise Hay, Susan Jeffers, Ph.D., and Caroline Myss, Ph.D.)

Menopause and Beyond

Mother-Daughter Wisdom

The Power of Joy

The Secret Pleasures of Menopause

Women's Bodies, Women's Wisdom

Inside-Out Wellness (with Dr. Wayne W. Dyer)

A DAILY DOSE OF WOMEN'S WISDOM

DR CHRISTIANE NORTHRUP

HAY HOUSE

Carlsbad, California • New York City • London
Sydney •Johannesburg • Vancouver • New Delhi

First published and distributed in the United Kingdom by:
Hay House UK Ltd, Astley House, 33 Notting Hill Gate, London W11 3JQ
Tel: +44 (0)20 3675 2450; Fax: +44 (0)20 3675 2451; www.hayhouse.co.uk

Published and distributed in the United States of America by:
Hay House Inc., PO Box 5100, Carlsbad, CA 92018-5100
Tel: (1) 760 431 7695 or (800) 654 5126
Fax: (1) 760 431 6948 or (800) 650 5115; www.hayhouse.com

Published and distributed in Australia by:
Hay House Australia Ltd, 18/36 Ralph St, Alexandria NSW 2015
Tel: (61) 2 9669 4299; Fax: (61) 2 9669 4144; www.hayhouse.com.au

Published and distributed in the Republic of South Africa by:
Hay House SA (Pty) Ltd, PO Box 990, Witkoppen 2068
info@hayhouse.co.za; www.hayhouse.co.za

Published and distributed in India by:
Hay House Publishers India, Muskaan Complex, Plot No.3, B-2,
Vasant Kunj, New Delhi 110 070
Tel: (91) 11 4176 1620; Fax: (91) 11 4176 1630; www.hayhouse.co.in

Distributed in Canada by:
Raincoast Books, 2440 Viking Way, Richmond, B.C. V6V 1N2
Tel: (1) 604 448 7100; Fax: (1) 604 270 7161; www.raincoast.com

Copyright © 2017 by Christiane Northrup, M.D.

The moral rights of the author have been asserted.

Cover design: Amy Grigoriou; Interior design: Pamela Homan;
Photo of Dr Northrup: Bill Miles

The information given in this book should not be treated as a substitute for
professional medical advice; always consult a medical practitioner. Any use
of information in this book is at the reader's discretion and risk. Neither the
author nor the publisher can be held responsible for any loss, claim or damage
arising out of the use, or misuse, of the suggestions made, the failure to take
medical advice or for any material on third party websites.

A catalogue record for this book is available from the British Library.

ISBN: 978-1-78817-027-7

Printed and bound in Great Britain by TJ International Ltd, Padstow, Cornwall.

MIX
Paper from
responsible sources
FSC® C013056
www.fsc.org

To all who have awakened to the reality
of the inner wisdom that is always guiding us—
body, mind, and spirit.

PREFACE

Getting your daily dose of women's wisdom by reading one or more of these quotes every day can become an important part of your health care. Why? Because what you pay attention to expands. In a world in which women are taught to focus on all the things that can go wrong with their bodies, here is your solution: a daily reminder about everything that can go right. And the more you focus on what can go right and why, the healthier you will become.

This isn't just some fluffy idea. It is the way your brain and body are designed to work. There is a part of the brain stem known as the Reticular Activating System (RAS) that takes what you focus on and creates a filter for it—screening out what's not important and enhancing what is. This happens automatically. It is why, when you decide that you like a certain kind of car, for example, and spend a bit of time learning more about it, you start to see that car everywhere. Or when you learn a new word you've never heard before, you start hearing it everywhere.

When you begin your day with a dose of the women's wisdom found in this book, your reticular activating system will begin to go to work on your behalf. You will start to observe and experience your body—and its processes—in a different way. You will begin to *trust* your body and its processes, becoming far more likely to experience everything that is going right with your body. Because of the spell that is contained in uplifting words and thoughts, you will find it much easier to tap into the innate wisdom that lives in your cells. Think of your daily dose of women's wisdom as both a nutrient to enhance your health and an immunization against negativity. And most of all, enjoy taking in the ideas contained here. They are the result of nearly four decades of experience on the front lines of women's health as an ob/gyn physician. And all have stood the test of time.

Dr Christiane Northrup

You are an ever-renewing,
ever-changing, ever-growing being,
born with an inner guidance that
helps you create and maintain
vibrant health and happiness.

To create health today, look at yourself in the mirror—especially at the parts you don't like—and say, "I accept myself unconditionally right now." Expect critical thoughts to arise, and accept them too. In 30 days, your body image will be transformed.

Rejoice in your inner guidance, knowing
that it's always available to lead
you to maximum health and fulfillment.

The Law of Attraction is the most powerful law in the universe. It states that like attracts like. Your thoughts and emotions create an energy field around you that draws people, places, and events to you that match your own vibratory rate.

Ninety-five percent of the beliefs
and thoughts creating your reality are
unconscious and inherited from your
parents and their parents before them.
The 5 percent of you that can change that
unconscious programming is your conscious
mind. This is where your hopes and dreams
live. To improve your health and life, you
must, literally, change your mind—both
conscious and unconscious.

Write down everything you want in life. Then take off the brakes. What would it be like to let your creative talents or your true self manifest fully? By writing your desires down, you'll be able to identify and change the limiting beliefs that are blocking you from accomplishing all you can do and be.

If anything were possible—quickly, easily, and now—what would your life look like? Who would be in it? What would you be doing? Where would you be living? What would you look and feel like? Invite your future self into your present to help you become the person of your dreams.

Today and every day, use the positive
power of your thoughts to consciously
create a healthier and more delightful life.

Thoughts are an important part
of your inner wisdom—and they are very
powerful. A thought held long enough and
repeated often enough becomes a belief.
A belief then becomes your biology.
Beliefs are energetic forces that create
the physical basis for your individual
life and your health.

Your decisions about medical treatment
are not irreversible. Because your body
is constantly changing and evolving,
it's a good idea to review and update
your approach as your body and
circumstances change.

Listen to your heart today.
Feel your feelings fully without judging
them. Emotions are your guidance system.
If you allow yourself to feel all your feelings
fully, regardless of whether they're sad,
angry, or joyous, your heart's
wisdom will heal your pain.

No one can fix your life for you.
You need to set out consciously to
do it for yourself. You must trust what
you know in your bones: your body is your
ally, and it will always point you in the
direction you need to go next.

There are many ways to heal.
Eventually, any externally imposed
guidelines for how to become well
must be consistent with your own inner
guidance system. You must learn to
support yourself through self-respect,
not through restrictive regimens filled
with *shoulds* and *oughts*
that feel punitive.

When faced with a dilemma, take a
moment to sit with the issue. Don't rush
to decide what to do. Intend to let Divine
inspiration flow to you, and it will be so!

The next time you get an ache or
a pain, soften the area around it with
compassion. Ask your body what it needs.
Listen deeply for the answer.

When you can clearly state what you want and why, you are instantly in alignment with your inner guidance. In doing so, you also have the capacity to acknowledge what you don't want!

You build your state of health every day through your thoughts, beliefs, emotions, and behaviors. Your cells believe every word you say!

If you could consciously appreciate the things that need to change in your life, you wouldn't have to create physical conditions to get your own attention. Common chronic symptoms often signal that it's time for you to let go of someone or something in your life that no longer serves you.

Nothing will change in your outer circumstances until you learn to value your own life and your own gifts as much as you've been taught to value and nurture the lives of others. Service through self-sacrifice (martyrdom) is a dead-end street.

Release resentment and anger
regularly after allowing yourself to feel
these emotions fully. Do this by saying, "I
now forgive and release [fill in the blank].
I let loose and let go, and I am free." Once
you begin, you'll find more and more things
to release. This practice is a powerful way
to rejuvenate your body and your life.

Know that depression is
anger turned inward. When you allow
yourself to feel your anger, resentment, and
disappointment, your energy is mobilized,
and you'll find that you're on your way to
better health. Have the courage to feel
uncomfortable emotions so that you
may release them when it's time.

The path of true abundance comes
from spending time, thought, and energy
on those areas of your life that are most
fulfilling to you. Over time, this is how
you create the life of your dreams.

In order to rediscover your authentic
self and break the cycle of self-sacrifice,
follow your heart. When you're asked to do
something for someone else, say no or say,
"I need some time to think things over.
I'll get back to you." In this way,
you proactively cultivate a loving
relationship with yourself.

The inability to love and accept yourself and your humanity is at the heart of many illnesses. To be loved and accepted, you must start by loving yourself. If you have traits that you consider unlovable, you must love them anyway—it's a paradox.

The more you move toward what
makes you feel good, and move away from
those things that bring you distress and
pain, the healthier you will be.

You are an individual who is part of a greater whole. The best way to express the Divine part of yourself is by becoming all of who you are. Your body directs you toward full personal expression by letting you know what feels right and what doesn't. Illness is often a sign that you need to make an adjustment in your life path.

Go to a bookstore or library and use your inner guidance to help you make a choice. See which book speaks to you. Acknowledge that you have the wisdom to choose the right reading material at the right time. You can't make a mistake.

Your beliefs go much deeper than your thoughts. Think of your mind as an iceberg. The conscious part peeks above the surface. The submerged part, the biggest section, is the so-called subconscious. It's important to understand that your beliefs and memories are actually biological constructs in your body, and so you can't simply will them away.

True health begins with your thoughts. Thinking about comfort, strength, flexibility, and youthfulness attracts those qualities into your life and body. Dwelling on illness, fear, disease, and pain does just the opposite. Your work is to notice and change your thoughts and move them in the direction of health and happiness.

Dreams reveal the beneficial and nonbeneficial directions you're focusing your energy toward and how and where you need to make adjustments. So keep a notebook beside your bed, and before going to sleep, write down a question you'd like answered. Jot down your dreams first thing in the morning and share them with a trusted friend. Over time, you'll find your solutions . . . and your memory and intuition will improve.

Ultimately, you must be willing to take responsibility for your life if you are to truly create health. This means understanding that illnesses have meaning. They don't just jump out of the closet and land on you.

Regret about things from your past is natural. But failure to work through the emotion keeps your cells locked in that earlier time, so you can't create anything new in the present. Feel your regrets fully, shed your tears if necessary, love yourself for them, and then let them go!

You've been told that hard work and discipline are the keys to a successful and healthy life. This is only part of the truth. Being willing to receive the best of what life has to offer is also a crucial skill.

Problem-solving is entirely different from creating health. To enjoy increased well-being, make a paradigm shift to a new way of thinking about your body, mind, and spiritual connection with the universe.

Your immune system is strengthened by the number of supportive relationships you have in your life. Studies have shown that those with the most varied social support networks are the least likely to get colds!

Your body and its condition is a barometer that's always trying to tell you in which direction to go for maximum creativity, health, and fulfillment. Repeat this often: "Because I am human, I get off track sometimes, but I can always get back on."

Do you have a clear sense of purpose?
Do you acknowledge that as an individual
you have the power to create your life,
while simultaneously acknowledging the
larger forces at work in the universe? Do
you understand the paradox of knowing
that you can influence many events
but you can't control everything?

If you want to have world peace—peace
in your town, peace in your family, and even
peace in your bedroom—simply begin with
whatever creates peace within you.
This vibration will emanate from you
in waves, which will have a very
positive impact on the world.

Your task isn't to kill the messenger of your illness by ignoring it, complaining about it, or simply suppressing your symptoms. Your task is to examine your life with compassion and honesty and identify the places that are crying out for love, acceptance, harmony, and fulfillment. Your body is nothing but a field of ideas, so make sure that those ideas represent your best interests.

When there's a conflict between the intellect (what you think) and the heart (what you feel), the heart always wins. But sometimes the feelings of the heart become translated into symptoms or illnesses so that you're forced to stop and experience them fully.

Your midlife years are a time for you to complete some of the tasks you started in adolescence. Now is the time to grieve the loss of any unrealized dreams from the past and prepare your body for the next stage of your life. When you dare to do so, you'll find that you're ready for the springtime of the second half of your journey.

Midlife is a call to "wake up from the family trance." To thrive, you just let your soul take the lead from here on out.

You know what it's like when you
have a bad day. You have an argument, get
cut off in traffic, miss an appointment—it's
a snowball effect. You can prevent that by
pre-paving. Set your intent for a joyous,
fulfilling day first thing in the morning
before you leave the house. Visualize it
for a few seconds, and then step
out in happy anticipation.

Many women have a natural thinking process that is circular and multimodal, not linear and causal. Ideas, thoughts, and wisdom come from all your parts: your brain, your uterus, and your Higher Power. You must learn to trust all aspects of your intelligence, not just your intellect.

Practicing gratitude regularly is a powerful way to receive more of what you really want, including vibrant health.

Your body is a symbol of your whole
life, who you are, and what your soul is like.
You co-create your physical self through
the laws of science as well as
through the laws of Spirit.

The processes of death and birth
are very similar. The difference is . . .
who is waiting on the other side.

Imagine your sexuality as holy and sacred,
a gift from the same Source that created
the ocean, the waves, and the stars.

It is essential for your health to find a few things every day that you really appreciate. You can choose mundane things: your shoes, the face of a good friend—even a clean bathroom in a gas station. The more you appreciate, the more you'll attract good things into your life, including optimal health!

At midlife more than at any other
time, you have a renewed opportunity
to reinvent yourself and fuel
your life from Spirit.

The heart has an electromagnetic
field that is 60 times larger than the
electromagnetic field of the brain. When
you feel love and appreciation in your
heart, your heartbeat stabilizes—and this
energy enlivens and heals your entire body.

When both you and your partner commit to taking 100 percent responsibility for your roles in your relationship, you can create magic! This is exciting and very beneficial for your health. On the other hand, it's also possible for one person to change the dynamics of a relationship in a positive way.

Remember that deciding to be happy
and healthy requires courage and focus.
It is ever so much easier to allow
negativity and fear to run your life.

Maintain a healthy level of sexuality
throughout your life by making pleasure a
priority that you plan for. This need
not include a partner.

Sex is a form of nonverbal communication
that strips the ego's defenses bare. To have
a good sex life, you must first appreciate
and love yourself. You must also be willing
to accept pleasure and let go of anger.

Although it's been said that "home is where the heart is," it's also true that this is where the heart most easily gets broken. Heal your heart by coming home to yourself. This is a lifelong process that involves opening up more and more to all your feelings.

You have the capacity to remain strong, attractive, and vital in mind, body, and spirit throughout your entire life. Deterioration with age isn't inevitable.

The processes of conception, gestation, labor, and birth are physical metaphors for how Spirit comes into matter and how creation comes into being. You are here to give birth to the highest and best that is waiting to be born through you.

Express the truth of whatever
you're feeling. Go into it and make the
sounds you need to make and cry or
yell as long as necessary. When you stay
completely within your innermost self, you'll
often discover that your body—through
weeping, moving, and making sounds—has
the innate ability to heal painful
memories from your past.

All your creations, including your children, have a life force of their own. In order for them to reach their full potential, you must eventually release control over them and let them go!

If a word or phrase continually comes
to mind, it's important. It has meaning.
Explore it, write about it, and meditate on
it. Accept it without judgment, knowing that
its significance will become clear eventually.

Sometimes your body can heal if you
will simply give yourself permission
to listen to its messages.

Your body doesn't know the
difference between what's real and
what you're thinking about and imagining.
Every thought is a biochemical reality in
the body. Uplifting ideas and emotions
are associated with an entirely different
mix of neuropeptides and hormones
than those of panic, fear, or anger.
So entertain thoughts that produce
the biochemistry of health and joy.

No one can make you angry without
your permission. Accept that your anger is
yours and that it's telling you something you
need to know. The next time you get angry,
ask yourself, *What do I want that I'm not
getting? How can I go about getting it by
using my own power in concert
with the power of the Divine?*

Only one part of who you really
are exists in a physical body. The rest is
outside of time and space. It is your Higher
Self. And it is always guiding you.

As a woman, your task is to learn, minute by minute, to respect yourself and your body, including all its wondrous processes.

As a woman, it's important for you to regularly spend time in settings where only women are present. When women gather together, each holds a piece of the whole story. In the early stages of self-awareness, women often don't tell the whole truth if there's a man in the room; we have been socialized to tailor our conversations to accommodate the other gender.

When your motivation for doing something comes from a positive place, you'll find a deep well of physical energy within you to sustain your efforts.

To create the highest and best that is within you, you must constantly let go of the old and welcome the new.

A health-care provider can have
all the credentials in the world and still be
the wrong person for you. You have the
ability to determine whether a doctor is
right for you by trusting your gut and having
the courage to seek a second
opinion if necessary.

It's possible to work consciously
with your dreams because they're a
powerful part of your inner guidance
system. The more you commit to
remembering and working with
them, the clearer they'll become.

Seek outside help if you need it. We
live in a society that promotes the myth of
the rugged individual who needs no one.
Seeking help, including therapy, isn't a sign
of weakness. It's a sign of strength to
allow others to help you.

As you read this, consciously relax your shoulders, neck, and back. Take a full, deep breath in and out through your nose. This simple process uplifts and energizes you and metabolizes stress hormones.

Your body was designed to move and stretch regularly. Incorporate regular movement into your daily life for optimal health. Why not start by dancing around your kitchen while preparing meals or cleaning up?

Ask yourself this question: *If I only had six months to live, how would I spend my time now?* Don't wait. Start spending your time that way today and every day.

No matter what has happened in your life, you have the power to change what that event means to you and thus change your experience, both emotionally and physically. Therein lies your power to heal.

A good therapist should be like a
midwife, standing by while you
give birth to the best in you.

When you sincerely invite in the Divine (your inner guidance, Higher Power, or Spirit) to assist you with your life, you're granting permission for your life to change. Those areas that no longer serve your higher purpose may start to disintegrate. This is scary—and also cause for celebration!

Regardless of where you begin to
reclaim and explore your sexuality,
it is helpful to know that female sexuality,
by its very nature, can be a total
sensory experience involving
your whole body and soul.

At midlife, you find yourself questioning the value of many of your relationships, including those you've never dared to look at too closely before. What you'll often discover is that many of your relationships (whether they be with your partner, your relatives, or your friends) need updating.

The life force that enlivens us is powerful, and life is big! Regularly release the past and prepare to be surprised and delighted by life.

Rather than think you need to go
on an archaeological dig into your personal
history, just look at your life in the present
moment to see what your past
beliefs have created.

Intimacy can take place only in a relationship that is a partnership, not one based on intersecting dependencies.

Much of the pain of any illness comes
from your own perception of its meaning.
When someone you respect tells you they
understand and that "it's not all in your
head," that affirmation can give you hope
and remind you that all illness—including
broken bones—is associated with physical,
mental, and emotional factors.

Whatever choices you make in life,
there will be consequences. Saying
yes to one thing always involves saying
no to another. Enlist your gut instincts
to help you make the right choices.

Your body was created to move
toward the people, places, things, and work
that bring you the most joy and pleasure.
You're designed to move away from what
brings you sadness, fear, and anger. In other
words, your body works better in states of
joy and anticipation. It doesn't work well
when you're feeling bad or don't
like what you're doing.

Loving everything about yourself—even the parts you consider unacceptable—is an act of personal power. It is the beginning of healing.

When you stop fighting those who
are there to help you, it's quite a relief.
Giving yourself permission to let another
individual support you can be a
profoundly healing experience.

Learn that it's good for you to stand up for yourself at the first sign of discomfort in a relationship. This is the best way to avoid being a victim.

You can contribute positively to the redefinition of aging by remaining youthful and vibrant throughout your life. This process starts with your beliefs about getting older. You can change the beliefs that no longer serve you at any age.

Regardless of what you believe about spirituality, it's important to bring a sense of the sacred into your everyday life. Your spirituality is in every part of you; it's not something that's set aside for special days in special buildings.

In a true partnership, both members are equally powerful and equally vulnerable. In such a relationship, you can allow yourself periods of intimacy offset by time alone. You may find that you thrive on a balance between separateness and togetherness.

The next time you start having a
bad day, stop everything and notice what
you've been thinking. Bring yourself into
the present moment. Touch the fabric on
your clothing. Run your hand over a smooth
surface. Breathe fully. Choose one thing
to be grateful for. This simple process
normalizes blood pressure, heart rate,
and breathing—and will turn a
bad day into a good one.

Commit to believing in yourself.
Someone has to make the first move.

When you pour out your
heart to another and feel your
humanity and vulnerability, the
floodgates of healing open.

Pay attention to whether you're using exercise to run away from your feelings or as a way to decrease stress. It's much better to deal with the source of the issue than to use a workout as a fix.

If you have a headache every Monday morning when it's time to go to work, perhaps you're driving the wrong car, taking the wrong route, or working in the wrong profession or at the wrong place. Take time to figure out the message.

Life is a buffet of endless choices.
When you say yes to something, the
universe lines up a whole new path. But
that yes also means saying no to other
possibilities. Staying stuck in ambivalence
because you're afraid of making a choice
leads nowhere. Take a chance.
Say yes to something.

Chronological age is how old you are on your birthday. Biological age is how old your body is physiologically. After about 35, these two "ages" may have little in common. It's possible to be "35" when your chronological age is 60 or beyond.

Your power to heal and stay healthy works
best in the present moment. When you're
truly present, you can heal almost anything.
Living in the now is a skill that you develop
through introspection, meditation, and
taking leaps of faith into freedom and joy—
one small leap at a time, one day at a time.

Intuition is the direct perception of truth or fact, independent of any reasoning process. Your inner guidance responds to your own or another's energy field through intuition, an ability you were born with. You were probably highly intuitive as a young girl, and you can remember and strengthen your intuitive intelligence through conscious, consistent use.

Nurturing others at the expense of yourself can set the pattern for ill health. You deserve everything that you also wish for others.

Nothing is ever just in your head.
Nothing is ever just in your body.
They are intrinsically linked—always.

This civilization hasn't done a good job
with the energy called delight and joy. Yet
these emotions are the very essence of life
and direct your inner guidance to
bring abundance into your life.

Vibrant health and a sense of
humor will make you very attractive
and sexy, regardless of your age!

Respect, care for, and love the
body you have. Vow to treat yourself and
your body with kindness even though there
may be some aspects of yourself
you don't really like just yet.

Are you willing to give up revenge
or the belief that the experiences you've
had in life should have happened to you in
a different way? To do so, you have to ask
for help from your inner wisdom
or your Higher Power.

Women with good friends live the longest.

At midlife, you no longer have the wiggle room to abuse yourself the way you did in your 20s. At this point, either you start to enter the springtime of the second half of your life or you begin to deteriorate. The choice is yours.

Your body is a barometer of truth. The beauty of the truth is that it's always refreshing and you never get tired of it.

Time alone in a natural setting is often a catalyst to connect with your spirituality. Find a tree, rock, or special place to wake up your senses. Allow the power of nature to heal you.

Appreciate the fullness of your
feminine intelligence, which comes not
just through your intellect but also through
your body's cycles. Your feelings are
also part of your intuition.

Commit to living your dreams one day at a time. Through this process, you heal yourself, your family, your community, and your planet.

Thoughts and positive emotions that
are held for 15 seconds or more without
contradiction begin to attract their physical
equivalents. Use this to your advantage by
focusing your mind and emotions on how
you'd like to feel right now, not what you'd
like to avoid or are angry about.

Rather than asking the universe to fulfill a shopping list created from your ego, surrender your desires to the Divine within, which already knows—often better than you do—what will be most fulfilling for you. Just say, "Okay, Higher Power"—or Divine Beloved or God—"bring it on. I'm ready to receive my Highest Good."

Forgive yourself for everything you didn't know in the past. Don't waste any of your precious energy beating up yourself or anyone else. Your power to change your life is in the present, regardless of your past.

A large part of creating health—or anything else, including wealth—is learning how to take in praise and allowing yourself to feel success and completion physically. If you don't practice receiving in this way, you're motivated only by thoughts such as: *There's so much more to do; I'll never get it all done.* This is a health risk. Take praise, accomplishments, and achievements into your heart regularly.

Caring for yourself isn't self-indulgence;
it's self-preservation. This might be a
radical notion for you, as you may
have been taught that self-sacrifice is
synonymous with being a "good" woman.
Have the courage to care for yourself.

You have to give your body credit
for its innate wisdom. You don't need to
know exactly why something is happening
in order to respond to it. Understanding
comes after you've allowed yourself to
experience what you're feeling. Healing is
an organic process that happens physically
as well as in your emotions. In fact,
the intellect is the last part of
you to get the message.

If you don't heed the messages
from your body the first time they're
delivered, you'll get hit with a bigger
hammer the next time. A delay or denial
requires your body to speak louder and
louder to get your attention. The purpose
of emotions, regardless of what they are,
is to help you feel and participate fully in
your own life. Stop and experience them!
Then change your behavior accordingly.

Think of your physical self as the outward manifestation of your mind. There will never be another you. That's because your body is shaped moment by moment by the kinds of thoughts that you're having on a day-to-day basis and what you look at and concentrate on.

Celebrate every relationship you've ever had. For better or worse, your relationships are your best teachers. And on a soul level, you've attracted each and every one of them so you can learn and grow.

Understand that humans are wired for ecstasy. Make it a regular part of your life, in whatever way pleases you, as long as it doesn't bring harm to others.

Make a habit of noticing what's
working in your life and appreciate it
and receive it with gratitude. Accept all
compliments graciously. Receive comfort!
Receive support! Receive joy!

It takes far more courage to
notice the positive than the negative.
You've been conditioned by your culture
and the mainstream media to focus on what
could go wrong instead of what's working
well. What you pay attention to expands,
so have the courage to remain positive
whenever possible.

Get in the habit of noticing and
writing down everything you want—no holds
barred. What kind of car would you like?
What sort of clothes? What type of house?
Whom do you want to be with? Be playful.
The universe is very creative and often
delivers in ways that exceed
your expectations. Trust it.

Our culture doesn't always
believe that creativity is valuable for its
own sake. To be considered worthwhile, an
activity must be associated with tangible
rewards or productivity and money.
Happily, it's possible to be creative
and prosperous at the same time.

At least three times a day, stop
whatever you're doing for 30 seconds,
put your hand over your heart, and do a
gratitude and appreciation "check-in." Bring
to mind someone or something you love
unconditionally, such as a dog or young
child, until a warm feeling envelops
your heart and chest.

Perhaps you need to rephrase the question from *What purpose does my illness serve?* to *What's the illness that will serve my purpose?* Sometimes you have to get sick in order to secure a socially acceptable reason to rest.

You're meant to create and grow and change. In order to do that, you sometimes have to go through discomfort.

Resolve to understand the dynamics
of health and money. Spend your money
on things and activities that bring you the
most fulfillment, and spend less money
on the "stuff" that will ultimately
have no meaning to you.

The right path always feels too
good to be true. It always feels like so
much fun that you can't believe it. When
you're following that route, your body
works well and you also feel your best.

Through writing, you can learn that your thoughts are deeply connected with your "feeling self." Every word that comes to mind will have meaning, which is connected to your entire being. Write as often as you can, even if it's just one sentence at a time.

Your inner wisdom will instruct you if you have a problem. You must then ask yourself, *What do I have to lose if I solve the problem right now?* Better yet, *What do I have to gain if I solve the problem right now?*

Grieving and learning to trust
again are major issues following loss.
You must stay with what you're feeling and
give yourself time to mourn your loss.
Grief is not self-indulgent. It is a
necessary step toward health.

When you feel upset or stressed, take
a "time-out" to breathe. Simply take
a few moments to focus on your breath
rather than on any negative thoughts.
Breathing fully in and out through your
nose engages your "rest and restore"
parasympathetic nervous system. This
quiets your mind and calms your body.

Opt for optimism. Studies show that those who see the glass half full actually live healthier, longer lives. Remember, being positive is a choice that also takes courage.

Studies have shown that women in
their 70s who continue to learn new
things physically and mentally (which always
involves a bit of discomfort at first) have
the same mental capacity as shown
on brain scans as 20-year-olds.

Holding in negative emotions such as grief and anger is exhausting. Naming them and releasing them regularly through writing, movement, tears, singing, or making sounds frees you up to live a full, vibrant life.

Unresolved childhood pain is a risk factor for disease, medication use, and premature death. Thankfully, it's easy to heal this pain as an adult. Just go inside and love that scared little kid on a regular basis till you grow her up!

Think of your social network as your immune-system safety net. At some level, every human illness is connected with a lack of social support. Thus, it behooves you to look at your life and ask yourself how many different types of people are in your safety net. Remember, no man or woman is an island. You are a member of a herd species.

The purpose or function of an addiction is
to put a buffer between yourself and your
awareness of your feelings. An addiction
serves to numb you so that you're out
of touch with what you know and feel.
Recovery is the process of feeling fully
and truly coming home to yourself.

Be extremely selective about what you allow into your environment. Your central nervous system was never meant to process all the bad news from around the world—set to dramatic music on the evening news! Being choosy about what you let into your life is a skill that's acquired over time.

Forgiveness is a health practice.
It has nothing to do with condoning the
behavior of the person you need to forgive.
Nor does it mean that that person should
be allowed into your current life. Instead, it
is a decision to finally free yourself from
the entrapment of resentment and
anger and the health consequences
of these toxic emotions.

Adopt the attitude that everything that happens to you—especially if you've been hurt or wronged—has a reason that you sometimes can't see. Be willing to go along with it and be as gracious as possible. Sometimes you have to accept the unacceptable. When you do so, your cells won't suffer and neither will your immune system—and you'll feel a lot better!

Rejoice in the knowledge that you
have the inner power to create
Heaven on Earth in your own life.

Making a commitment to healing involves
two steps: the first is admitting that healing
is necessary, and the second is opening
yourself to the information that you begin
to attract following the acknowledgment.

If you don't allow yourself to eat
something you want, it's likely that your
desire for it will increase to uncomfortable
levels. Eat just a little of what you crave
during the day. If it's chocolate, go for the
good stuff. Make it an event and
savor it slowly and fully.

Wounds don't heal until they're witnessed. If you're stuck in denial, your secrets will remain locked in your cells, unavailable for witnessing and healing. Past wounds mend whenever you're ready to acknowledge and then release them.

The biggest fear for many is that
of abandonment. This can create all kinds
of immune system problems because this
system is greatly influenced by your sense
of safety, security, and belonging. Enhance
your immune system function by accepting
yourself for exactly who you are
right now, this very minute.

Perhaps you're looking for a
source of endless nourishment that
will let you know that you're okay, that
you're worthy. Ultimately, the only one
who can connect with this source is you.

You were born with a unique passion
and purpose. And that may be as simple
as deciding to be happy! When you're
fulfilling this purpose, you contribute
to the health of the entire planet.

When you allow others to exploit,
judge, and control your innate gifts and
talents, you put your health at risk.

You betray yourself when you become
overcommitted to *doing* at the expense
of *being*, and *thinking* at the expense
of *feeling*. When you acknowledge the
validity and beauty of your inner world,
you empower the feminine aspects of your
being and bring them into balance with
the masculine. As a result, your heart
opens and your health improves.

For an intimate partnership to work—
regardless of gender or sexual orientation—
one member needs to embody the yang
masculine energy, which wants respect.
And the other needs to embody the
feminine yin energy, which wants to be
cherished. Decide which one you are.
You can't have it both ways if you want to
maintain balance and chemistry sustainably.

What did you love when you were
between 9 and 11 years old? Sometimes
what you have to do—if you've been talked
out of who you really are—is to go back
and ask a sibling, parent, or other relative,
"What was I like? What did I love to do
at that age?" The answer holds the
key to your deepest fulfillment.

You have a Divine spark within you,
and your body is permeated and nourished
by spiritual energy and guidance. Having
faith and trust in this reality is an important
part of creating health. Ask for guidance
and be open to receiving it.

You can look at the glass as half empty or half full. And the minute you start looking at it as half full, all the glasses around you start to fill up. This seems simplistic, but it's the way the Law of Attraction works. Focusing on what's full will bring more good things into your life!

Your entire concept of "the mind"
needs to be expanded considerably.
The mind can no longer be thought of as
being confined to the brain or the intellect.
It exists in every cell of your body. And
even beyond your body. Every thought you
think has a biochemical equivalent. Every
emotion you feel has one as well!

Forgiveness is an experience of grace, a gift you give yourself. The most challenging person to forgive is usually yourself.

The bond between mother and
child is the most intimate one in human
experience. Love, welcome, and receptivity
at the beginning of life greatly enhance a
child's health and happiness throughout
her lifetime. Fortunately, it's always
possible to "re-mother" and love oneself
unconditionally at any age, thereby
enhancing health and well-being.

Anyone who has the courage to live
joyfully and pleasurably despite a history
of abuse, neglect, grief, or disappointment
is actually contributing to the health and
healing of the entire planet. It isn't selfish to
be happy and fulfilled. It's essential if you
ever expect things to change for the better.

Once an experience is consciously named and internalized, physically and emotionally, it becomes real for you in a new, more potent way. Creating optimal health involves naming your experiences for what they are—whether joyous or painful—and then remembering that the forward thrust you need for your life is within you right now, regardless of your past.

Creativity is your birthright. It
shows up best when you consciously
decide to allow it, notice it, nurture it, and
create a structure to contain and manifest it
physically. That structure might be a
two-hour writing period each day, a
30-minute meditation, or journaling
your dreams every morning.

The next time you feel fear, anger,
grief, despair, or sorrow, simply allow
yourself to experience the emotion without
attaching a story to it. Open your heart
to it, knowing that this can lighten it while
your mind cannot. Love yourself for all the
feelings you judge as "bad" or "negative."
Notice your love and acceptance shift,
change, and relieve these emotions.

There are events in your life that
can't be explained or changed, so just
acknowledge them; feel them; and release
the rage, guilt, loss, anger, and grief. This
process takes time and attention, and
it can heal your body and your life.

You leak energy in any situation in which your anger or fear is controlling your ability to move forward. Simply notice who or what you're thinking, worrying, or obsessing about. Accept yourself for this, then gently shift your focus to your senses. Feel the wind on your face, listen to a train in the distance, look at a tree, or just feel the fabric of your clothing. Coming to your senses frees the mind and stops the "gerbil wheel" spinning in your head!

When you change your life for the better in any way, your entire family benefits. You set the tone. The well-being of the family and of society itself depends upon women becoming and remaining healthy. So you owe it to yourself to put yourself first and take the time you need to heal.

Joseph Campbell said that you must be willing to get rid of the life you had planned in order to have the life that is waiting for you. Remember this when you're having a hard time letting go.

Tears, movement, and sound are
part of your emotional digestive system.
These things help release blocked energy
in the body. Moving through pain by
feeling your way through it is "the
pain that ends the pain."

Consciously notice the quality of your thoughts as they arise so that you know where you are right now. If you know where you are, then you can do a better job of choosing where you must go.

Take time to make a list of all the
aspects of your life that are working
and another list of those that need to
change. Ask for Divine guidance to alter
the things you're willing to change
now. Then take action!

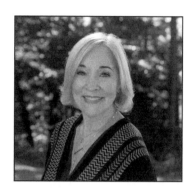

ABOUT THE AUTHOR

Dr Christiane Northrup, board-certified ob/gyn, former assistant clinical professor of ob/gyn at the University of Vermont College of Medicine, *New York Times* best-selling author, is a visionary pioneer in women's health. After decades on the front line of her profession as a practicing physician in obstetrics and gynecology, she is now dedicating her life to helping women truly flourish by learning how to enhance all that can go right with their bodies. Dr Northrup is a leading proponent of medicine that acknowledges the unity of mind, body, emotions, and spirit. Internationally known for her empowering approach to women's health and wellness, she teaches women (and many men) how to thrive at every stage of life and encourages them to create health on all levels by tuning in to their inner wisdom.

As a business owner, physician, former surgeon, mother, writer, and speaker, Dr Northrup acknowledges our individual and collective capacity for growth, freedom, joy, and balance. She is also thrilled with her company Amata, whose name is derived from the Thai words for "ageless" and "eternal." This company is devoted to creating and distributing products that contribute to vibrant health and well-being throughout the life cycle (www.amatalife.com).

When she's not traveling, Dr Northrup loves devoting her leisure time to dancing Argentine tango, staying fit through Pilates and resistance stretching, going to the movies, getting together with friends and family, potluck dinners, boating, process painting, and reading.

Dr Northrup stays in touch with her worldwide community through her Internet radio show, *Flourish!*, as well as Facebook, Twitter, Instagram, her e-letter, and her website, www.drnorthrup.com.

Hay House Titles of Related Interest

YOU CAN HEAL YOUR LIFE, the movie,
starring Louise Hay & Friends
(available as a 1-DVD program, an expanded 2-DVD set,
and an online streaming video)
Learn more at www.hayhouse.com/louise-movie

THE SHIFT, the movie,
starring Dr. Wayne W. Dyer
(available as a 1-DVD program, an expanded 2-DVD set,
and an online streaming video)
Learn more at www.hayhouse.com/the-shift-movie

*HOLY SHIFT: 365 Daily Meditations from A Course in
Miracles,* edited by Robert Holden, Ph.D.

*MIRACLES NOW: 108 Life-Changing Tools for Less Stress, More
Flow, and Finding Your True Purpose,* by Gabrielle Bernstein

*UPLIFTING PRAYERS TO LIGHT YOUR WAY: 200 Invocations
for Challenging Times,* by Sonia Choquette

All of the above are available at www.hayhouse.co.uk

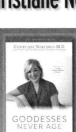
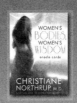
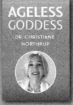

NOTES

NOTES

NOTES

NOTES

NOTES

NOTES

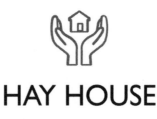

HAY HOUSE

Look within

Join the conversation about latest products,
events, exclusive offers and more.

f Hay House UK

🐦 @HayHouseUK

📷 @hayhouseuk

❤ healyourlife.com

We'd love to hear from you!